Surviving Tarlov
Resource and Recovery Guide for Tarlov/Meningeal Cyst Surgery

Sheryl Bacon Jones

DEDICATION

To my fellow sufferers of Tarlov/meningeal cysts, I hope this book brings you hope, faith, and the empowerment you need to get to the other side.

CONTENTS

ACKNOWLEDGMENTS

There have been many helpers along my path that were indispensable to the process and I owe a great deal of my life to them. To my impossibly perfect husband, Damon Jones, who carried me back and forth to the bathroom, fed me, comforted me, and carried the burden of all that was left in my absence. To my loving daughter, Lumen, who cared for and comforted me and never made me feel bad about all the things I could not do with her during this ordeal. For my Mom and Dad, Chip and Pennie Bacon, who helped me find strength to carry on, helped us to not lose everything we had in the process, and always believed I would recover. To my sister and her husband, Ginnie and KaRon Williams, who ignored my requests and drove all day long to get to me just so they could hold my hand while I cried. To my father-in-law, Charles Jones, for being our partner in life and always doing everything he can to help us. To Brad and Elizabeth Jones, who made the long journey with three kids to setup a Christmas tree in our living room so that Lumen could feel normal for a while. To my sister-in-law and brother-in-law, Amber and Chris Hart, for setting up a secret GoFundMe page to help pay for my surgery. To my beautiful ragdoll, Zeus, who taught me it was possible to have a beautiful life just laying around and never leaving the house. To my good friend, Brenda Morgan, for introducing me to Kris Carr. To my amazing co-worker and friend, Allison Bennett, for restoring my faith in God's helpers. To Allison Halquist, for helping me to realize my own strength against internal fears and anxieties. To Iben Larrsen, for helping me believe I would get better and giving my life meaning again. To Dr. Bradley Fullerton, who helped get me into remission the first time and offered me free treatments for months trying to help me out of my pain the second time around. To Dr. Scott Simms, for helping me get off Vicodin and always taking the time to share his wealth of knowledge on all things holistic. To Dr. Tiffany Jones-Lee for being the first doctor to really listen to me and help me figure out what was wrong. And for Dr. Frank Feigenbaum who ignored the naysayers and forged ahead in his quest to help Tarlov/meningeal cyst sufferers live a normal, happy life. You are all angels sent from God and I am forever grateful for each and every one of you.

Disclaimer: I am not a doctor. This information is of the "hard knock" variety that comes from desperation and Google endurance marathons. I have tested almost any natural remedy you could imagine for this situation and have narrowed down what I have found to be useful into this guide for you. I do not include suggested supplement amounts because I am not qualified to do so. I can tell you it is often a much higher dosage then is listed on the bottle. For this reason, I highly recommend you seek out a holistic doctor in your area that can really help you to heal, not just mask symptoms. If this is a new healthcare area for you, allow me to suggest a few words to use in your Google marathon: functional doctor, naturopathic doctor, holistic doctor, nutritionist. It is most useful to have advice on supplement amounts, nutritional support, access to specialized treatments, and a professional who genuinely believes in your ability to heal.

Introduction

There comes a time in all our lives when we must come face to face with our greatest fears. Perhaps, it is the loss of a loved one, a job, or a house. For us, it came in the form of a loss of our physical abilities, intense pain, and a loss of identity changing everything about who we were and how our lives functioned. A Tarlov/meningeal cyst diagnosis is one of the hardest diagnosis to receive and even harder to deal with. This disease forces us into great periods of suffering and even greater moments of fear when we must face what is and take steps towards reclaiming our lives.

You may not yet realize it, but you are on a great journey. This is the beginning of your David vs. Goliath quest. This book was written to remind you that you will win. You will be strengthened by this journey in more ways than you can realize and your life will be transformed in more ways than you can even comprehend at this moment. I have been steeped in the same fears, worries, and doubts as you. I have missed years of life staring out a window contemplating why I was born and what the point of all my suffering was. In my reflections, I have found meaning and hope. The dark that surrounded me could not survive the light within me and neither can yours.

This is my story and a compilation of the resources I found to help me through to the other side. Your story may look different and lead you down different paths. I can only hope that in reading one story of triumph, you will awaken to the story of triumph within you. This disease is the fire that burns us to ashes and overcoming it causes us to fly as the risen phoenix. I do not know you, but we are tied together because of our shared suffering. I feel as you feel. I fight as you fight. I love as you love. We are all striving to return to the place of comfort where we once lived. A place where our biggest concern was getting our kids to gymnastics on time or losing ten pounds before our high school reunion. I am here to tell you that you may never return to the life you once had. You will instead create an entirely new world for yourself and it will be magical beyond your wildest dreams. However, you must go through the fire first. I hope you find this book useful and that it may serve as part of your arsenal against what you face.

Chapter One
My Story

The year 2009 was a life changing year for me. I was finally moving in a solid direction with my career and relationship. My husband, Damon, and I had just got married in February and we were over the moon happy. I was 25 at the time and we had been living on my parent's property while we all built an online business from the ground up. It had been years of pinching pennies, sharing a car, and struggling to make a place for ourselves in the market. By this time, we were well on our way and making enough money to sustain ourselves. Unfortunately, I was also a heavy drinker. I binge drank in college and the terrible habit followed me well into my twenties.

On one July night, I went to use the restroom and it would change the entire course of my life. It was dark and I was drunk. My parent's enormous bloodhound laid directly in front of the closed bathroom door. I tripped over her and my foot searched for ground on the other side, closest to the door. Because the door was closed, it did not open and allow room for my next step, so my foot was forced into a blunt right angle. I heard a loud pop inside my right hip and limped into the bathroom. I had to slowly lower myself onto the toilet because it felt like I could not bend my hip very easily. I stumbled out to Damon and joked, "I think I just messed myself up!" I laughed and made another whiskey and Pepsi. My life would never be the same again.

The disability came on slow. Six months later, Damon and I finally had enough income history with our business that we were approved for a house of our own. We excitedly moved all our stuff, including an antique fridge up some stairs. I was overcome with a searing pain in my lower back and hip. My pelvis felt swollen and tender. I had to lay on the floor while Damon finished moving things on his own. I knew something was wrong, but I had no idea of the severity or what I was about to face. I called a local doctor and was lucky enough to get an appointment right away. The doctor diagnosed me with SI Joint Dysfunction. He gave me strong anti-inflammatories and told me it would heal on its own with time. I popped the pills for ten days as I was instructed, and I recovered…for a little while.

I would continue to have episodes of pain with increasing frequency. I began the merry go round of doctor visits that included medical doctors, chiropractors, gynecologists, sports doctors and occasional desperate trips to the emergency room. I had a new diagnosis to go with each new doctor, all of them leading to prescriptions of pain pills and anti-inflammatories. One sports doctor told me that I simply needed to exercise through the pain and it would take care of itself. I went home that day and did an exercise program. I remember vividly my hip being in intense pain and instead of stopping, I started beating on my side in frustration trying to force it into submission. The pain became a permanent fixture without intervals of relief from that period forward. I found that I could not walk for even short distances without searing pain in my lower back and pelvis. I returned to him and he said they had found an ovarian cyst in a scan and I should go to a gynecologist to see if that was the issue. When I was with the gynecologist, he stated there was no way my pain was from a cyst and it was probably just ovulation pain! He suggested I learn to live with it. When I replied that I could not live this way, he simply stated, "Well, then kill yourself." Everything went blank in that moment and I hung my head and cried in utter despair while he began to back pedal and make it seem like it was a good natured joke we were meant to have a good laugh about. When I returned home and called the sports doctor once more for help, he would not even take my call or allow me to set an appointment. I could have remained incredibly angry about this, and do not get me wrong, we did turn the gynecologist into the medical board (although nothing ever came of it). However, in hindsight, that doctor did me a real favor. He taught me that I had to be responsible for my own health.

It was up to me to find the answers and reject the nonsense. It was then, that I began to realize that conventional medicine was not going to rescue me on its own. I became bedridden and completely depressed.

I am not one to roll over, so after some time to emotionally recover from this experience, I began seeing a local chiropractor and was put through the litany of rolling, stretching and popping. One day, a lump of inflammation appeared over my sacrum, which would stay with me for a decade. The inflammation alerted my chiropractor to a bigger issue and so finally, an MRI was ordered. When my results came in, I was so excited to receive an actual diagnosis, however the look on my chiropractor's face did not reflect the same excitement. She grimly told me I had a large Tarlov cyst in my sacrum and that there really was not a consensus on the best treatment. I went home, began researching, and finally understood the scope of what I was dealing with.

There was not a lot of information about Tarlov cysts available at the time and doctors who performed the surgeries were just beginning to make any kind of headway. For me, surgery was not even an option anyway. One of the caveats to being your own employer is that you do not get insurance unless you pay an exuberant amount for it. We did not have insurance. I could not afford the surgery out of pocket and I was too scared to get the risky surgery at the time, even if I could have. I became determined to find another solution.

Enter Kris Carr. One of my trusted friends had seen Kris Carr talk about her journey with stage IV cancer on *Oprah*. I watched Kris's documentary, *Crazy, Sexy Cancer*, and was hooked. Those who were following her protocol showed great progress and their tumors were shrinking. In my mind, if a tumor could shrink, so too could a cyst. However, my line of thinking was faulty because I did not realize that a Tarlov/meningeal cyst is not the same thing as a regular fluid filled cyst found elsewhere in the body, such as a breast cyst (Refer to

Chapter 2). Either way I had a plan and that was all I needed to get some hope back. I bought her book *Crazy, Sexy Diet* and I began the 21 day protocol outlined in the book.

At that time, I had been bedridden for six months, only leaving for doctor appointments with the use of a wheelchair. By the end of month seven, something miraculous happened. My constant pain ceased. I could not believe it! I still experienced great pain if I walked more than a very short distance, but at least I could sit without pain, which meant I could begin to think properly again. It also meant that I could stop taking the massive amounts of pain pills and anti-inflammatories I was on, which caused me mental disturbances and increased depression. An important part of my personal journey also coincided, in order to follow Kris's diet, I quit drinking. I would struggle to quit completely for the next decade, but I would eventually overcome my addiction.

The great decrease in my pain from simply changing my diet was astounding to me. Apparently, I knew nothing about nutrition or how the body worked prior to this experience. I honestly thought being skinny meant you were healthy. My intake was Lean Cuisines and diet Pepsi and I thought I was doing pretty good. This food revelation blew my mind wide opened and all sorts of new ideas flooded into my life. I had already discovered that mainstream medicine could not help me (outside of surgery) and so I began to turn to alternative doctors and medicine.

I spent thousands on crazy treatments that involved chelation shots into my throat and ears, blood cleansing, where a huge amount of my blood was taken, cleansed and pumped back into my body. I was put on well over 35 supplements a day and my life revolved around taking them. Upon reflection, much of this was extreme, expensive and likely unnecessary. My doctor at the time, after months of expensive treatment without recovery, finally determined that the issue was in my hip and sacrum (no kidding) and that I needed Prolo

Therapy (an injection of sucrose that irritates the old injury and stimulates renewed healing efforts by the body).

I began getting regular weekly treatments and to my extreme delight, saw leaps of improvement. However, if I deviated from the diet or did too much, the pain and dysfunction would return with a vengeance. I was still a prisoner in my own body and I wanted freedom. I was finally able to walk further and further and was no longer wheelchair bound. I can remember the day I realized recovery was possible. Damon and I had gone to a festival and reluctantly left my wheelchair in the car. I walked and walked without pain! I looked at him and just burst into tears. We cried and held each other as people pushed past us and kids screamed with delight from the top of the Ferris wheel. It is a moment that is seared into my memory with the addition of fireworks shooting off in the sky around us. Four years after it had all begun, Damon and I decided I was recovered enough to have a baby.

I got pregnant and went to Austin to have a much more intensive treatment called Platelet Rich Plasma (PRP) Therapy (they inject the site with your own platelets to speed healing). I wanted to alleviate as much pain as I could before the baby began to grow and I would face the physical feat of labor. It worked and I was mostly pain free! I could do whatever I wanted within reason. I still had minor flare ups with over exertion, but it no longer hindered my life. I was elated. I had an incredibly painful natural childbirth and got one more PRP injection afterwards, thinking it would prevent a possible repeat of dysfunction. I continued with my life, being careful to avoid certain movements, for the next four years.

My daughter, Lumen, is incredibly active and loves to dance. I wanted to be able to dance freely with her and so I made a fateful decision… I would go back in for one more PRP injection so that I could recover all the way. Recovery is not what happened. Something was immediately different following my PRP treatment this time.

When I stood up from the table a burning pain traveled all the way down the front of my right leg and into my foot. I had never had leg or foot pain before and I was in for a real shock.

The recovery period for PRP is six weeks and then you begin to see the full effects of the treatment. A few weeks into recovery, I knew something was very wrong. The level of intense nerve pain was unbearable. I could not get out of bed and I began to panic. One morning, in desperation, I got out of bed and began screaming and yanking curtains off the wall. I picked up a turquoise mother elephant statue that I had always loved and smashed it into a million pieces before falling to the ground in pain. It was if I was trying to tell God that I had already lived through this nightmare once and I could not go through it again. Little did I know, the nightmare was going to be taken to new levels that would break me down to my very core.

Damon has a family cabin in Austin and so we decided to move into the cabin "temporarily" while I went back to my PRP doctor and tried to fix whatever had gone wrong. The time spent in that cabin over the following months was likened to being dropped into the burning pit of Hell. To this day, I have not yet returned to the scene of the crime and often have flashbacks. Suffice to say, the me that went in, was not the me that came out.

My symptoms were far worse than ever before. I was relegated to laying completely flat, without even the slightest elevation (I would remain this way for well over a year). Damon had to keep me covered in ice at all times and I could often be heard screaming "Ice! Ice!" from the room. I would regularly suffer from patches of frostbite and developed a persistent bed sore. Damon had to carry me to the bathroom and bathe me while Lumen watched on. My bowels did not work properly and the number of pills I was on meant I had to do a water enema every single day, sometimes multiple times without much result. Eventually, Lumen would no longer ask me to play or make her a snack. The hardest part was hearing her play outside the window or crying out for Daddy when she needed comfort. I was in the deepest of despair.

I contemplated death every second and researched ways to do it every day as I lay in bed staring at the ceiling. I even asked Damon to hide his gun, which was unnecessary because I couldn't even get out of bed to grab it if I wanted. Thankfully, the maternal instincts within me would not allow me to let Lumen go through the loss of what was left of her mother. I hoped that I could somehow recover the way I had before with the use of food. I spent months laying in that cabin waiting for food to fix what it could not.

Eventually, my PRP doctor realized the treatments were not helping and ordered another MRI. I barely made it through, but in the end, I had a clear picture of what I was up against this time around. The cyst was enormous and completely filled my sacrum. There was no amount of green juice or PRP treatments that was going to be able to rectify this.

We were fortunate to have insurance now and so, with my doctor's recommendation, I began the process of meeting with Dr. Feigenbaum (one of the only doctors in the United States who treats Tarlov and meningeal cysts). I got an appointment within a month and made the painful trek to Dallas. Dr. Feigenbaum informed me that I had a large, 2-3" meningeal cyst that had erupted out of my spinal sac into my sacrum. The cyst had broken through the top of my sacrum, eroded away nearly all of my bottom vertebrae, and had completely crushed all of the nerves that run the bottom half of my body. Surgery was pertinent and he put me on the list. I was absolutely terrified and forced to find coping mechanisms that continue to serve me today, which I will share with you in this resource guide.

I had my surgery on August 21, 2018, a little over nine years after this journey began for me. Recovery was beyond slow. I remained completely bedridden for at least six months post-surgery and I continued to be relegated to bed consistently as flare ups would occur at the drop of a hat. I was on six Vicodin a day and had trouble feeling positive about my outcome and I felt recovery would not come again. I was a member of a Facebook Tarlov group, but my fears were so intense that I could not bear to read about other's fears, worries and doubts. The stories of recovery mentally hurt me as well, because others were recovering their physical capabilities far faster than I was and I thought this meant something about my ability to fully recover. I was still deeply depressed and suicidal, so I found a therapist who agreed to meet with me weekly on Skype. She refused to let me think I would not recover and helped me to focus on releasing all the shadows that were coming up. She gave me weekly assignments that I would pour my focus into, rather than wallowing in my grief. This was a huge turning point for me mentally and helped me to begin solidifying some of the lessons that I had learned and to find meaning in my circumstances.

At the six months post-op mark, I was able to be out of bed for 10 minutes or so and could walk a little bit, but I would not be able to sit for a very long time to come. I made the decision to discontinue the Vicodin. Not because I no longer needed it, but because I needed to find my inner strength to pull myself out of the hole I was in and Vicodin was only digging me in deeper.

I began to experience leaps of improvement every few months and my faith and hope were slowly restored. This was not a quick process and improvement could include something as simple as being able to bathe myself or make a snack without help. It would be well over a year and a half before I could begin to sit longer than a handful of minutes or go to the grocery store with my family. I am now just over 26 months post-op as I write this, and I continue to improve. I can drive, play with Lumen in the park, cook dinner, make love to my husband, sit in most chairs for long periods of time, and I can walk all day long with little discomfort. What the body is able to achieve with enough time is simply astounding. My flare-ups use to last months, then weeks, then days, and now hours, if that. I follow Kris Carr's diet with some modifications and have created a combination of protocols that I follow specific to nerve healing. I am happier than I have ever been. I am more grateful then I have ever been. I can live my life freely.

I am not fully recovered yet. I still have some pain and setbacks and limitations. Running is mostly off the table and there is no way I could make it through a Zumba class (to be fair, I could not make it through a Zumba class before this happened!). However, because of the immense suffering I survived, I no longer have the same mental limitations. Lying flat on my back in such an extreme state of suffering for so long was like a death of sorts. The Sheryl that was there before died into something that only experience can describe. Going through this opened a dimension within me that I did not know existed, a place where I am good enough as I am and I am strong and capable of facing challenges with grace. I have been shown what is important in life and almost more importantly, what is not. I have been completely transformed by this. My cyst has been the greatest teacher in my life and as hard as it is for me to even believe, I am grateful for it. I know you may not find yourself in a place of gratitude just yet, but know someday you will. You are meant for something incredibly special. That is why you are going through this. You must allow it to change you. One day, you will look back and see the dissolution of the old you and realize that you have now been reborn as an empowered individual with the strength to care for yourself, help others, and create a life of great meaning and joy.

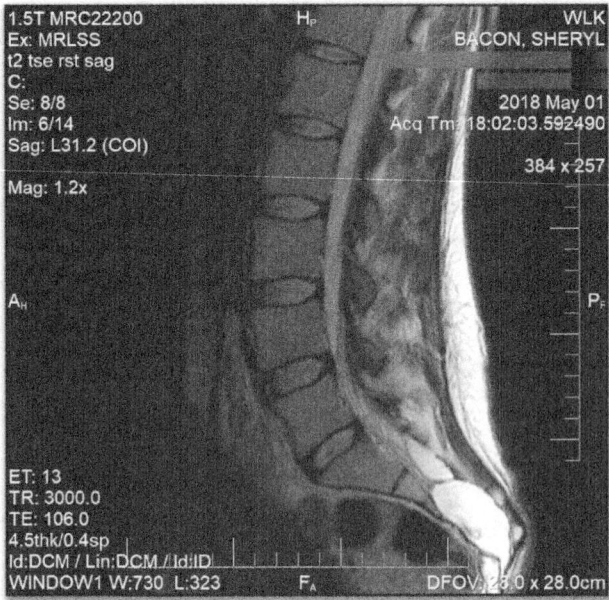

Sheryl Bacon Jones, MRI Scan
May 2018

Chapter Two
Tarlov Cysts vs Meningeal Cysts

While doing your research or reviewing potential doctors when considering your options, you may have come across two terms: Tarlov Cyst and Meningeal Cyst. A meningeal cyst is a cerebrospinal fluid filled cyst. Both the meningeal and Tarlov cysts are meningeal cysts, however the Tarlov cyst is innervated. This means that a Tarlov cyst has formed out of the actual nerve sheath itself and is a part of the nerve structure. A general meningeal cyst (that is not innervated, hereafter referred to as a meningeal cyst) forms out of the actual spinal sac encasing the spine. Depending on the location of the meningeal cyst, it can be almost impossible to tell the difference between the two until the surgery is performed. However, size is a good indicator. They both exert pressure on surrounding nerves and can create the same incapacitating symptoms to the individual. Common symptoms include, but are certainly not limited to:

- Sacral or tail bone pain
- Sacral pressure
- Pain with sitting, standing or walking
- Pain in the legs and feet
- Pain in the hip or hips
- Leg weakness, tingling, or numbness
- Bowel or bladder dysfunction
- Sexual dysfunction or pain
- Vaginal, pelvic, anal and/or abdominal pain
- Headaches

Tarlov cysts are smaller and multiple are generally found in the patient. Removing a Tarlov cyst does not necessarily mean it will not return and the patient may need to have more than one surgery to address these cysts over their lifetime. A meningeal cyst tends to be much larger because it makes use of the larger surface area of the spinal sac and once removed it does not return. This is a bonus; however, it has the potential to cause more widespread damage due to its size.

Sufferers of both experience comparable symptoms and they are often found in the S1-S4/S5 region of the spinal canal. There have been instances of these cysts being found in the lumbar, thoracic and cervical spine, because they are able to form wherever there is a nerve root along the spine. However, those are rarer. There is much speculation as to what causes these cysts, which is outside the scope of this resource guide. Suffice to say, once you have experienced one, the primary goal is relief.

Treatment for these cysts has been developed quite slowly because they were long thought to be asymptomatic. In fact, you may still face many health professionals that refuse to believe these cysts could be causing your symptoms and therefore obtaining a correct diagnosis can be difficult, if not almost impossible for some. For this reason, insurance companies are also inconsistent in their coverage. Fortunately, knowledge in this area is growing due to the dedicated doctors who recognize the validity of this disease and work tirelessly to find solutions for sufferers.

In the past, many types of treatments have been utilized with varied success. Draining the cyst proved to be a temporary solution as the cyst simply fills back up. Fibrin glue has been injected, with the aim being to seal off the cyst from refilling. However, complications from fibrin injections have been cited frequently enough for it to fall out of favor and is no longer the recommended approach. Surgical removal is fast becoming one of the more successful treatments. As more patients go this route, more data is being produced to support this treatment. Recovery from the surgery is extensive and incredibly long. However, the alternative is potentially a lifelong affliction. So, for many of us, surgery becomes our best and only option.

Chapter Three
Pre-Surgery

The decision to have surgery is not an easy one. The process for surgery involves opening the sacral, cervical, lumbar, or thoracic spinal cavity (referred to as a laminectomy) and then the cyst/s are treated and/or removed. In the case of a sacral laminectomy, a small portion of the sacrum is removed in order to gain access to the cyst/s. This portion is then reconstructed with an absorbable plating, which will dissolve and be replaced with scar tissue over a one-two year period. I have seen variations on the material used to replace the sacral section. The main thing for consideration is the process used for addressing the cyst/s.

The whole procedure is completed with the assistance of nerve monitoring and aided with a microscope to ensure that other nerves are not disturbed or damaged. It is a major surgery and there are risks involved. It is up to you to determine if the risks are worth it. For me, personally, I feel I had no choice. My meningeal cyst was extremely large, I was completely disabled, in a level of pain that could not be managed, and damage was being done to my structural system.

The great news is that we are facing this diagnosis at a time where treatment is becoming more readily available to us. I cannot help but think of those that suffered from this in decades past when diagnosis and treatment had not yet been developed. We are truly fortunate that we have solutions available to us. Part of your solution will likely be finding a surgeon to perform your operation. It is vitally important to recognize that not all doctors are created equal. This is a fairly new treatment and it is important that you locate a doctor with extensive experience treating cysts in such fragile locations within the spine. You do not want a doctor poking around in there that is unfamiliar with the procedure. Finding the right doctor may mean you will need to travel for the operation. According to The Tarlov Cyst Disease Foundation's website, the following doctors are suggested:

United States

Feigenbaum, Frank, M.D. (Neurosurgeon)
Dallas, TX

Schrot, Rudolph J., MD MAS FAANS (Neurosurgeon)
Sacramento, CA

Henderson, Fraser C. Sr. M.D. (Neurosurgeon)
Silver Spring, MD

Canada

Murphy, Kieran M.D. MB FRCPC FSIR (Interventional Neuroradiologist)
Toronto, Ontario

Europe

Zollner, Georges, M.D. (Interventional Neuroradiologist)
Strasbourg, France

Marcettini, Paolo, M.D. (Neurologist with specialty in Pain Management)
Milan, Italy

South America

Arantes, Aluizio, M.D.
Brazil

NOTE: *This information is subject to change. Verify information as needed.*

Most often, you can send in your medical records and your MRI for an evaluation over the phone. This is an important step whether you have the surgery or not because it gives you more information about your options. There is a chance that the doctor feels your issue is not Tarlov/meningeal related, in which case you can explore other options. If you and your chosen doctor feel that your issue is the cyst/s, then you can proceed from this point and get yourself on the waiting list.

Once you have decided on surgery, selected your surgeon and set a date, you will most likely face some fear and anxiety about your impending surgery. I certainly did. I have suffered from anxiety and panic attacks to varying degrees throughout my life and I can tell you this was a whole new level of angst. I was faced with a subjectively lengthy wait before surgery, so I had to find coping mechanisms to get me through. My biggest helpers were:

Surgery Meditation
Guided meditation for the purpose of surgery and any other medical procedures has been scientifically proven to decrease anxiety, decrease post-surgical pain and recovery time, as well as, reducing the need for medication and even lowering blood loss during the procedure. The meditation I used is from Belleruth Naparstek with Health Journeys called *Guided Meditation for Successful Surgery*. This meditation is award winning and has been researched and proven effective by prestigious health institutions such as the Cleveland Clinic, Penn State, UC Davis and Blue Shield of California.

I had an experience related to my use of this meditation just prior to surgery that convinced me of its power. During the meditation, Belleruth suggests that your blood will be slowed for surgery, making the procedure go more smoothly. While I was in the surgery prep area the nurse drawing my blood was shocked at how slow my blood was moving and stated that he had never seen anything like it. There are other meditations available on Health Journeys' website that cover areas of pain and post-surgical healing. Check them out and see if any of them interest you.

The Untethered Soul by Michael Singer

This book focuses on mindfulness and shifting your perspective on how you view yourself and your thought patterns. It helps you to put some space between yourself and your fears so that your strength can grow. It offers methods that can be applied to scary emotions and helps you to settle yourself. There are many books that cover this topic, but Michael has a real gift of explaining things clearly. This book was imperative to me for facing my fears and anxieties over surgery and recovery in general. I cannot recommend this book highly enough for transforming your life overall.

Nature Therapy

If you are like me, you feel trapped in your bed. In my case, I could not just lay or sit anywhere. I had to be laying down and whatever I was laying on could not be too soft or springy. Thankfully, my parents gifted us with an outside cushioned swing that would fold out into a bed. I would lay outside in the sunshine every day on it. I would listen to my surgery meditation, read in my book or simply gaze at the trees and birds carrying on as if nothing was wrong. I found this to be deeply peaceful and a necessary way to cope with the pressure I was under.

It is important to try and change your scenery up a bit and getting outside has the added benefit of Vitamin D. Science has proven that being in nature (and in some cases simply viewing pictures of nature) reduced blood pressure, muscle tension and the production of stress hormones.

Earthing is a term that refers to connecting our bodies into the energy of the Earth for balancing and healing. The idea is to make direct contact with the Earth's surface electrons with your bare skin. Multiple scientific studies have emerged confirming the benefits of Earthing, which are:

Neutralizes Free Radicals that are generated from inflammation, stress, cell damage, trauma, and environmental toxins.

Improves Pain Management and Stress by normalizing cortisol levels and calming the nervous system. The nervous system is an electrical system, thus the zapping pain that accompanies nerve injury. It has been shown that an influx of negative electrons from the Earth's surface switches the autonomic nervous system from the sympathetic (fight or flight) to the parasympathetic (rest and digest).

Improves Inflammation via the reduction of cortisol on the system, which then increases the strength of the immune system.

Water is a great electricity conduit and so walking on wet grass or alongside a body of water increases conductivity. There are also many products you could purchase such as Earthing sheets or shoes, however the best method is simply taking your shoes off and going outside. I was unable to walk very much for a couple of years so I would often lay on a mat on the grass and allow my bare feet to dangle off the end and into the grass. It is recommended that you Earth for 20 minutes, twice a day to reap the full benefits. This is considered an Environmental Medicine and I believe it should be utilized throughout your life.

Despite whatever various techniques you use to get to surgery, there is a good chance being there the day of surgery will heighten and seemingly undo all your progress. Surgery is an unknown and this tends to activate our fight or flight. I was in pure panic mode and it was obvious to my nurses. They addressed it quickly by administering something to relax my nerves. Hopefully, this brings you comfort to know that they will help you once you get there. My anesthesiologist was an angel and she held my hand and comforted me. After they rolled me into to the operating room, she gently placed the mask over my face and it was over. The amount of mental relief I had after waking up from surgery was enough to carry me through the trying first months of recovery.

Reducing Anxiety Prior to Surgery

Anxiety is nothing more than magnified fear. Your reason for being fearful may be legitimate, as in needing back surgery and having your nerves exposed and possibly dissected. Anxiety however, is generally an overreaction to the fearful situation. It involves creating stories in the mind that intensify and add to the fear that is already there.

Catastrophizing is a huge component of anxiety. Catastrophizing is the tendency to take a situation and turn it into the worst-case scenario without direct proof of that being the case. The reason anxiety can run rampant is because we do not turn to face it when it arrives. Opting instead, to run away from the uncomfortable feelings, either by distracting ourselves, self-medicating or trying to mentally convince ourselves that we are okay. When we mentally engage with anxiety, we feed it. We end up in an argument essentially trying to convince ourselves that we are both right to have the anxiety and wrong at the same time.

In my opinion, the solution is to desensitize the overreaction by turning to face the anxiety when it arises. You can do this by noticing when anxious thoughts or feelings begin to surface and then taking time to stop and be with the feelings. Place all your focus on the feelings being created by the anxiety in your body. Sit with it instead of running. Slowly, you will build up resilience to these feelings and you will realize that your focused attention is stronger than any fleeting emotion.

Another important aspect to this process is to try your best to remain internally silent while watching the emotions within you. Resist making a story up about the anxiety or justifying or arguing with it. Once you remove story making, you remove energy and the emotion will fizzle out. Combining these two techniques has been the only solution I have ever found that works to reduce anxiety effectively.

Addressing Concerns About Arachnoiditis

A common fear is that having the surgery will cause Arachnoiditis. Arachnoiditis is a rare condition where the arachnoid (one of the membranes surrounding the spinal cord) becomes inflamed and swells due to infection, injury or compression of the spinal cord. This is a very painful condition that enhances nerve pain greatly.

I wish to share my opinion on the matter, but must add a disclaimer that I am not a doctor and these are my opinions only. There is much speculation that the Tarlov/meningeal surgery will cause arachnoiditis because according to *The National Institute of Health*, 60% of Arachnoiditis cases result from complications from spinal surgery. Therefore, it is incredibly important you choose a doctor that is well experienced in this area. Barring any issues during and after surgery, I would like to point out that the other listed causes of Arachnoiditis includes spinal taps, steroid injections, and epidural injections.

Generally, pain management doctors force these injections on Tarlov/meningeal patients as part of the requirements to continue with your oral pain prescription. If these injections are a known contributor to developing Arachnoiditis, it only makes sense to assume that getting these injections regularly are a greater threat than we may attribute to them. I believe the likeliness of developing Arachnoiditis is more strongly associated with continued injections.

Additionally, these injections are counterproductive to healing and may even make things worse. A 2017 study conducted by the *Journal of the American Medical Association (JAMA)* followed the outcomes of knee arthritis patients who received repeated injections for two years, using either corticosteroids or a placebo. Patients given steroids typically saw no pain relief, and actually demonstrated an increased progression of cartilage breakdown in the knee joint. The placebo group had slightly better pain numbers but lost only half as much cartilage as those injected with actual steroids. There are a ton more studies coming out regularly that indicate that steroids are not only ineffective, but actually cause direct injury in the long-term. That is why it is so important we educate ourselves and not fall victim to the unvalidated opinion of those in authority.

For many though, these injections are not optional because the pain is too great, and we are at the mercy of our pain management doctors to prescribe medication that help us through. You could print out all of the data supporting the research done, showing the adverse effects of utilizing steroids and see if your doctor is willing to read it and work with you. However, the chances of simply being dismissed are high.

The solution I put forth is to do everything in your power to manage pain as naturally as possible. Ideally, you can utilize diet, supplements, over the counter medications and natural modalities to deal with your pain after your post-surgery prescription runs out. Or, if you are lucky, you can find a compassionate pain management doctor who understands your specific situation and does not force these injections as a stipulation. Alternatives will be discussed in greater detail in the **Pain Management section** of this resource guide.

Chapter Four
Post-Surgery

I read in my surgeon's testimonials that many woke up from surgery and had instant relief for many of their issues. Some, never even filled their pain prescriptions and went grocery shopping as soon as they were checked out of the hospital. I sincerely hope this is the case for you. However, it was not the case for me. The immense pressure in my sacrum was gone, but the pain and dysfunction were not. I had to seriously lower my expectations and throw out any sort of preconceived timeline for recovery and I suggest you do the same. Perhaps you will get better within weeks, but if you do not, it is important for you to maintain a healthy outlook. Given that the suggested time frame of healing from my surgeon is 2+ years, it is more likely that it will take some time for many of us to see results.

I did not see real life altering results until around the six month mark, and from there, improvement still continues every three months or so. It seems I will see no improvements for months on end and just as I begin to wonder if I have reached the ceiling for my healing capacity, improvement happens. I have learned that I must practice absolute patience with myself and not compare my progress to anyone else's. A beautiful lesson for life in general. The following resources helped me with my recovery:

Hospital Bed
I could not sleep in my regular bed anymore because Damon and I co-sleep with Lumen. I was scared she would flail in her sleep and end up kicking me in my sacrum. We were lucky to be able to rent a hospital bed for me to use in the interim. This bed allowed me to sleep without fear and it also had an adjustable back that would allow me to sit up once I was able to do so.

After I recovered enough to sleep in my regular bed, we moved the hospital bed into the living room so that I could go in there to do my work. It helped me to feel more normal to get out of my bedroom and have somewhere comfortable to go. Perhaps your insurance will allow you to rent one as well.

It is vital you find ways to change your scenery up however you are able. It lifts your spirits and keeps you more involved in the lives of your loved ones. Time away from family functions is inevitable before and after surgery and it can be a brutal pill to swallow. Creating new ways of interacting must be initiated, or else you may end up isolating yourself which is counterproductive to healing.

Average monthly rental cost is between $200-$500. Medicare does provide coverage if the bed is deemed medically necessary. Call your insurance provider to get more information prior to surgery.

The IceMan

The DonJoy IceMan machine is a little miracle. I read about it from other patients who had purchased the machine to help with post-surgery swelling. It is a small machine that you fill with ice and water and it circulates the cold water through a flat pad that you can lay on. I brought the machine with me to the hospital and my wonderful nurse kept it full of ice for me. I continued to use the machine for months after surgery and it helped tremendously to keep pain levels down and the healing process. Ice reduces swelling, which relieves additional pressure and decreases pain. This is the reason an anti-inflammatory diet also reduces pain all over the body. The average cost for The IceMan is around $120.

Picker Upper

This handy dandy tool will make a huge difference in your life. You can use these to pick up trash on the ground, retrieve your cane, grab items too high for you to reach and so much more. It helps you to not feel totally helpless. Although, sometimes I found that I needed a picker upper to pick up my picker upper. That is an unsolvable dilemma.

I tried a couple of brands and found the one I like most is the E-Z Reacher Pro Plus Reaching Tool. I still use it all the time to clean my house and pick up stuff in the yard. If you have children, this is a fun way to get them involved with helping you with tasks of daily living. The average cost for the E-Z Reacher is $20.

Human Help

There is no doubt about it, you are going to need someone to help you after surgery. Even if you recover quickly, there is going to be a fair amount of time where you just cannot manage things on your own. I needed help for at least a year with many everyday tasks. I am just now able to do most things independently. Even if you can just get someone to bring you meals or pick up groceries for you it will go a long way. There are tons of delivery services for all kinds of things these days. If you have the cash, do yourself a favor.

Things are going to be different during this time. You are recovering from a major surgery and your life has probably been turned upside down. You will need to let go of control and the sooner, the better. I struggled with the cleanliness of my house. Damon was caring for me, our daughter, picking up my slack at work, cooking all of our meals, keeping my ice replenished, grocery shopping, doing laundry, etc. He did not have the time or energy to keep the house as I had kept it before. I faced deeply ingrained feelings of embarrassment when someone would come to visit, and the house was in total disarray. I had to learn that it was okay to let things fall apart and to accept outside help. I let go of needing appearances to be perfect and learned to let them be authentic instead. I faced my incapability and accepted it. This was a huge lesson for me, and it can be one for you too.

Chapter Five
Pain Management

There is no greater transformer than pain, but that does not mean you do not need help to cope with it. The amount of pain that comes along with a Tarlov/meningeal cyst is incomprehensible to most people. Nerve pain is a different beast. Therefore, many protocols will likely need to be deployed. Narcotics are most useful at first, but at some point, you will need to wean off these medications or reduce the amount you take for true healing to occur. According to Dr. Montiero and Dr. Coppola in their book *Defeat Neuropathy Now*, the medications people with nerve pain are prescribed actually cause nerve damage.

Below, is a list of things I found that helped manage my pain. This list will overlap some with the things listed in the **Nerve Healing Protocol section** because healing helps reduce pain. The top three supplements in this list were recommended to me from my chiropractor and I found them to be incredibly helpful, especially when I was weaning off Vicodin.

Phyto UltraComfort from Pure Encapsulations
Phyto UltraComfort is a combination of herbs that are proven to assist with pain management such as White Willow, Indian Frankincense, Turmeric, and Devil's Claw.

Salicin-B IC by NuMedica
Salicin is a precursor to aspirin and helps with joint discomfort and mobility.

Proteolytic Enzymes
These little helpers target inflammation. It is important that you take them on an empty stomach. You cannot overdo it, so take as many as you like throughout the day.

Magnesium

Magnesium is essential for nerve function and it helps promote relaxation of the nervous system. In turn, your pain is reduced and your mobility can be improved upon. Magnesium also helps with constipation, so it will assist with the pain of going to the restroom and help with any back up issues caused from the prescription medications you are taking. I use time release pills and I take 2 teaspoons of Daily Calm to assist with bathroom issues daily.

Advil

Before all of this began, I never took any pills for anything if it could be avoided. In this situation, I found it could not be avoided. I still occasionally take an Advil if needed, especially around my menstruation, which increases my discomfort. I have tried Advil, Aleve, and Tylenol and I find that Advil is the only one that does the trick for me.

BioFreeze

I have tried almost every over the counter topical pain reliever there is. Allow me to save you some trouble, stock up on BioFreeze. It is incredibly effective at numbing pain.

Back Patches

The patches I found to work the best are the Salonpas Lidocaine 4% with Menthol. I tried capsaicin patches as a more natural alternative, however the capsaicin causes a burning sensation which does not pair well with the pain of burning nerves, in my opinion. I could use capsaicin now if I need to without the same issue because of my level of healing, but I would not recommend them if you are in the thick of it. It is worth noting that my pain level no longer warrants the use of a backpatch.

The IceMan

I mention use of this in the **Post-Surgery section** and it is equally useful for pain in general. Again, The Ice Man is a small machine that you fill with ice and water and it circulates through a flat pad that you lie on. Before I purchased this, I would simply use baggies of ice which would often burst and soak my sheets. I also encountered frostbite from using freezer packs. Using The Ice Man alleviates these issues and stays cold for hours. The use of this machine is incredibly helpful in getting you through a flare up while reducing your prescription medications.

Baths

Soak in a bath with 2 cups Epsom salt and ¼ cup baking soda often. The magnesium found in Epsom salt is extremely calming to your nervous system. Furthermore, hot water helps to ease your body and mind. I found that I looked forward to my daily bath more than anything because it gave me my only opportunity to get out of bed.

Chapter Six
Nerve Healing Protocol

This is the biggie. Perhaps, it is the whole reason you even purchased this resource guide. It is important that you realize that nerves can and do heal. I am not talking about completely severed nerves here (although studies are showing advancements in that area as well). I am referring to our specific nerve situation, which is flattened or sliced nerves that are still intact. There is a prevalent myth in our country that peripheral nerves are nearly incapable of healing and if we suffer nerve damage, we are almost certainly doomed to a life of symptom management. Please do not allow this misinformation to become your truth.

Our bodies are healing machines and they will never give up attempting repairs on our behalf. There have been stories of paralyzed people suddenly regaining the ability to walk after years of being incapacitated. Anything and everything are always possible. The following protocols are scientifically backed and proven to help with the repair of nerve damage.

B-Vitamins
B-Vitamins are water soluble organic compounds that collectively play a crucial role in body maintenance, tissue development and cellular function. B-Vitamins are especially important for nerve regeneration. This cannot be overstated enough. B-Vitamins are so important to your nervous system that being deficient in them can be a cause of nerve damage. Many studies and evidence have been gathered that directly correlates B-Vitamins with promoting nerve repair and accelerating nerve regeneration and function. There is some Vitamin B found in Nuphoria Gold (see below), however I take an additional B-Complex vitamin to cover my bases.

Alpha-Lipoic Acid (ALA)

Alpha-Lipoic Acid has been shown to have a positive effect on nerve conduction and reduced neuropathic pain. ALA is a biggie for nerve repair. A study called the *Sydney 2 trial*, showed a 52% decrease in the experience of neuropathic pain after only five weeks of supplementing at 600 mg a day.

Turmeric (Curcumin) and Ginger

These two anti-inflammatory powerhouses offer a one-two punch for nerve pain. They can help with tingling, numbness, pain and loss of function. Turmeric is thought to prevent chronic neuropathic pain from settling in.

You could take this as an additional supplement. However, I like to make a big batch of Turmeric Tea every few days. My whole family loves Turmeric Tea and I enjoy introducing it to guests. I was introduced to Turmeric Tea by Dr. Andrew Weil who was researching why the people of Okinawa, Japan have such a significantly longer and healthier life span than those living in other countries. He found that this was a traditional drink that was consumed regularly. I have tweaked his recipe to suit my taste and you can find it in the **Diet and Exercise section** of this resource guide.

Omega-3s

These water and fat-soluble fatty acids play an important role in supporting nerve density and signal transmission. They have also long been touted for their positive effects on brain health and development.

Vitamin D

The "Sun Vitamin" features an array of extremely necessary benefits to the body. For our purpose, it has been shown to reduce severe neuropathy. Being deficient creates neuropathy. I believe we are meant to be connected to and energetically charged by the sun. I take a spray Vitamin D every day and try to sunbathe daily with at least

50% skin exposure (weather permitting).

Fat (monounsaturated fats)
A 2019 study published in the *Journal of Neuroscience*, reported that a diet high in healthy fats may effectively reverse the progression of neuropathy and restore nerve function. One explanation for this may be that the myelin sheath that covers and protects our nerves is made from fat. It only makes since that increasing healthy fat intake would support healing of damaged nerves. Bring on the avocados, oil, and nuts!

Lion's Mane
Lion's Mane is a strong anti-inflammatory, antioxidant and immune boosting herb that research has found to help repair nerve damage by stimulating nerve growth factor (NGF).

Infrared Light Therapy
This is the big kahuna as far as I am concerned. Laser therapy has been around for a while and it is scientifically established that it promotes healing and regeneration. However, the lasers of yesterday were very expensive, primarily used by physicians, would get so hot that they would burn the surrounding skin of the wound being healed, and penetration into the body was superficial. This is where NASA comes into play.

NASA was performing some experiments with infrared light in space involving various plants. They found that the infrared light promoted faster growth in the plants that were exposed. During discussions of these experiments, NASA learned of the limitations of this therapy for humans and partnered to create LED Infrared Light Therapy that solved the previous issues. Plus, because of the LEDs, the penetration could now reach a depth of approximately 1.5" into the body. This opened the door for the healing capability of infrared to reach the masses and to be studied further by scientists.

A 2015 study called "Far-Infrared Therapy Promotes Nerve Repair following End-to-End Neurorrhaphy in Rat Models of Sciatic Nerve Injury" appeared in *Evidence-Based Complementary and Alternative Medicine, Vol 2015.* This study focused on assessing the efficiency of utilizing far-infrared in the treatment of severe nerve damage in rats. They concluded that far-infrared is "a novel and noninvasive therapeutic modality to improve motor function, accelerate recovery from sciatic denervation-induced gastrocnemius muscle atrophy, modulate the inflammatory process during sciatic nerve injury, and enhance nerve regeneration following end-to-end neurorrhaphy in a rat model of peripheral nerve injury. Future studies using FIR as a noninvasive treatment modality for various peripheral nerve diseases and injuries can lead to the wide acceptance and standardization of this innovative therapy in clinics." In my view, far-infrared is the most promising nerve healing modality to be discovered.

One of the top brands out there is Anodyne. It consists of four separate small rectangle pads that you can either strap on using Velcro straps that come with the system or you can simply place the pads where needed. I lay on my side and tuck them into my waistband for a sacral treatment and then I roll onto my back and place them along my groin. My system also came with a shoe that allows me to place the pads inside of it for a foot treatment. Initially, I would use my system off and on, all day long. I continue to use it weekly.

CBD Oil

CBD blasts inflammation and pain out while eliminating immune related oxidative stress which allows the body to heal itself better and creates a significant reduction in neuropathy symptoms. I originally began taking CBD Oil for anxiety (one dropper full a day) and I simply continued during my recovery. I have tried several brands and my favorite by far is Green Roads.

Water

Water is critical to your body in countless ways, but it is especially important for someone trying to heal and detox. Staying hydrated helps to keep inflammation under control and avoid triggering pain receptors. Plus, drinking lots and lots of water can help with constipation, which could be inadvertently causing flare ups. It is pertinent you continually drink water to help your body recover and flush harmful prescription toxins out as quickly as possible.

Nuphoria Gold and Nuphoria Blue
These are nerve healing specific compound supplements that include many of the above listed nerve healing nutrients. You can create your own supplement regimen as you see fit utilizing the list provided. I read a book written by the creators of Nuphoria, Dr. Montiero and Dr. Coppola, called *Defeat Neuropathy Now*. That is why I chose to purchase their products. I supplement on top of Nuphoria because I believe it is what is best for my recovery plan. Even if you do not purchase their products, it is necessary in my opinion that you read their book. The information offered is invaluable for building confidence and hope in your nerve healing endeavor. It debunks many myths about nerve healing and replaces it with science backed facts that serves to prove what is possible with the right mindset and protocol.

Note: Nerves take time to heal and there is no real shortcut. You cannot expect to begin a nerve healing regimen and see results right away. It is said that you will need anywhere from three months to over a year to begin reaping the rewards of your hard work. This is the task we have been faced with. We did not get to where we are overnight and we will not get out of it overnight. We are all in this for the long haul.

Inner Work
In spirituality, it is believed that all diseases or ailments are connected to a deeper spiritual ailment that must be addressed before healing can be complete. In honor of this view, I wish to postulate that perhaps our shared condition could be attributed in some way to

other shared aspects of our lifestyles.

For instance, I have struggled with issues related to anxiety, panic, people pleasing, inauthenticity and negative emotion suppression. Perhaps you face a great deal of inner pressure that is unique to your personality traits. All of these intense emotional and mental components have a direct effect on the nervous system and creates a great deal of pressure. Maybe this pressure is playing a part in the introduction of these cysts into our systems. You may have noticed, as I have, that the pain intensifies when you are agitated or in a state of fear. I believe for us to heal completely and become whole, we must work through these emotional issues and begin to live our lives more authentically and true to who we are. Emotional health undoubtedly aids in the healing process and this has been confirmed by countless studies.

Beyond the healing process, I believe it could also serve as a preventative tool which may influence the future development of cysts or lack thereof. This has not been proven, but I believe the proof will be presented in our own lives through our own efforts.

Chapter Seven
Diet and Exercise

Your body is a healing master. If you need proof of this, think about a time you cut yourself. It healed right up without a trace. Your body is constantly renewing, regenerating and healing itself every second of every day. Your body is capable of a level of healing that you could scarcely believe. In order to heal, your body needs a couple of things.

First, the physical impediment to healing must be removed, i.e. the cyst either needs to be surgically removed or perhaps one day a way of shrinking the cysts will be discovered. My brilliant PRP (Platelet Rich Plasma) doctor postulated that there was a kink higher up in the nervous system that was pressurizing the nerve and created the "blow out". He thought perhaps if the pressure could be reduced, then the cyst would shrink and the nerve could heal itself. We were working on this hypothesis while I was in Austin and before I knew I had a meningeal cyst (a Tarlov cyst sprouts directly out of the nerve whereas a meningeal cyst sprouts out of the spinal sac onto the nerves). It would be interesting to discover if this does in fact play a part in the development of Tarlov cysts though.

Second, the body must have all the supplies it needs to do the work of recovery. You cannot expect your body to build a new foundation without the materials it needs to do so. The materials, of course, are what you eat and drink. There are two very different healing diets out there for us to consider, vegan and keto.

I have read instances of people healing with the keto diet and it is a very popular protocol for Multiple Sclerosis and other autoimmune conditions. MS effects the nervous system and therefore it is thought to heal many issues related to the neurological system. The most popular system is referred to as *The Wahls Protocol*, discovered by Dr. Terry Wahls. For me, a strictly keto diet was just not feasible for a couple of reasons. It is heavy on animal products, especially organ meats, which does not appeal to me. When I was on this diet, I felt sluggish compared to my vegan diet. More importantly, it ranks as one of the worst diets according to the *2020 U.S. News and World Report* that is released each year. They state that the keto diet is "fundamentally at odds with everything we know about long term health". The report continues to state that it is low in nutrition, creates negative health outcomes, and alters the gut microbiome in ways that increases inflammation and impacts immunity and health. This does not mean that it may not be suitable for some conditions or for short term use as a medicinal diet to aid in recovery. I have researched this diet extensively and believe it has many valid points for the quest of healing. However, more studies need to be done to ascertain the safety of living on this diet long term for me to personally be comfortable staying on it. It is worth noting that I do not have an autoimmune disease either, so the best path for you may look differently than mine, based on your situation. Although, I do believe in Dr. Wahls' work and I have incorporated many of the things she suggests. I use recipes from her cookbook from time to time.

On the flip side, there is Kris Carr's Crazy, Sexy Cancer Diet. This diet is a vegan, whole food-based diet that is heavy in living foods (aka raw) and copious amounts of fresh green juice. The magic in eating or juicing raw food is that you essentially capture the life inside the plant and transfer it to your body. This is the synchronicity that is meant to occur between you and your food and drinks. Each morning, you begin with a green juice that kick starts your healing and gives you more vitality then you can imagine. The benefit to it being juiced is that your body does not need to go through the arduous task of breaking your food down before it can use the nutrients within to make repairs. I have found great success on this diet with tremendous pain reduction and increased overall well-being and energy levels. I believe if you follow this diet for at least a month, you will see a dramatic reduction in your pain levels whether you have had the surgery or not. The downside to this diet for me is that you can run into trouble when it comes to getting enough Vitamin B (which is essential for nerve health and repair) and I tend to be anemic (iron deficient) on this diet no matter how many vegetables and fruits I consume that are high in iron. Plus, I believe some animal protein and fats are helpful and crucial in the healing process.

Therefore, through personal experimentation, I have created a diet that primarily follows Kris Carr's *Crazy, Sexy Cancer Diet* 90% of the time and I incorporate clean, grass-fed or wild caught protein sources 10% of the time. What this looks like for me is a diet of mostly living foods with lots of green juice and smoothies, a few weekly meals consisting of meat without the fat drained off, lots of fermented foods, some bone broth, and limited grains.

I implore you to check out Kris Carr's *Crazy, Sexy Diet* book and follow the 21-day plan at the back, with the addition of some grass-fed meat if you feel called to do so. The book is chock full of all the science and research you need to get yourself going in a healing direction. In my opinion, getting your diet right is one of the most important factors in facing any challenging health issue. Plus, if you can follow a whole food, vegetable heavy diet and stick with it for the long term, you may very well be preventing yourself from having to go through further illnesses later in life.

It is important that you drop any guilt you may have been conditioned to have from eating large amounts of food. You will need to eat three meals a day, plus hearty snacks in between. Real, whole foods are sacred and should not be treated as an enemy, but instead as a gift that heals your body with every bite. I find it incredibly wonderous that everything our bodies need sprouts right out of the ground or lives off the stuff that sprouts out of the ground! Below are some of my favorite plant-based recipes to give you a taste, so to speak. I give credit for where I found the recipes; however, I have tweaked some of these recipes to suit my taste.

<u>Green Juice by Kris Carr</u>

1 Cucumber

5 Stalks of Kale

1 Small Green Apple

4-5 Stalks of Celery

5 Stalks of Romaine Lettuce

1" Ginger Root

Juice all ingredients in a juicer or blend and strain.

<u>Green Power Protein by Kris Carr*</u>

1 Banana, Frozen

½ Green Apple, Cored and Seeded

1 ½ Cups Nondairy Milk

2 Tb Hemp Seeds

1 tsp Maca Powder

1 Pitted Medjool Date

2 Cups Greens

Blend all ingredients in a blender.

<u>Inflammation Heavyweight by Kris Carr*</u>

¾ Cup Blueberries, Frozen

½ Cup Cherries, Frozen

1 ½ Cup Nondairy Milk

2 Tb Hemp Seeds

¼ tsp Cinnamon

1 Cup Greens

Blend all ingredients in a blender.

*I like to add collagen, trace minerals, and kelp to my smoothies for a nutritional boost. You can find all sorts of add ins to suit your needs.

Source: *Crazy Sexy Juice* by Kris Carr

Turmeric Tea by Andrew Weil

16 Cups Water
2 Tb Ginger Root, Grated
2 Tb Turmeric Root, Grated
Juice of 1 Lemon
6 Tb Agave

Combine water, ginger and turmeric in a large pot and bring to a boil. Simmer for 10 minutes. Add lemon juice and agave, stir well. Allow to cool in pot before straining while transferring to a large pitcher. Store in refrigerator and enjoy within 3 days for best taste. **Note:** Turmeric will stain anything it touches. This includes your counter, kitchen utensils, pitcher and you.

Chickpea Salad

2 Cans Chickpeas, Drained
1 Stalk of Celery, Chopped
1 Pickle, Chopped
¼ Cup Purple Onion, Chopped
½ Cup Vegenaise
2+ tsp Dill weed
Salt and Pepper to Taste

Smash the chickpeas in a large bowl with a potato masher and add all other ingredients. Mix together and chill. Serve with sprouted bread, in a tortilla, or put on top of a salad.

Portabella Pita

2 Whole Wheat Pitas
2 Lg Portabella Mushrooms
1 Lg Tomato, Sliced Thick
4 Cloves Garlic, Chopped
Handful Basil Leaves
1/3 Cup EVOO
Salt and Pepper to Taste

Combine EVOO with garlic and brush some of it onto both sides of pita bread; set the rest aside. Brown both sides of the pita in a skillet on medium heat. Remove and set aside. Add remaining EVOO and brown the mushrooms, for about 5 minutes per side. Remove and set aside. Season tomatoes with salt and pepper and grill for about 1 minutes per side. Assemble the pita by layering on tomato, mushroom, and basil. Drizzle with EVOO or flax seed oil. **Note:** Raw Milk Feta can be crumbled on the top if you are eating dairy.

BBQ Tortilla Pizza
2 Whole Grain Tortillas
¼ Cup BBQ Sauce
¼ Purple Onion, Sliced
2 Tb Cilantro, Chopped
½ Cup Beans

Preheat oven to 375 degrees. Assemble the pizzas by layering tortilla with BBQ sauce, beans, and purple onion. Bake on a cookie sheet until crispy, about 5 minutes. Remove and top with cilantro.

My Favorite Snacks
Hummus and Celery/Bell Pepper Strips/or Plantain Chips
Cashews, Walnuts, Pistachios, Pecans
Coconut Yogurt with Sliced Bananas, Pumpkin Seeds and a Drizzle of Agave
Kale Chips
Trail Mix
Olives
Apple Slices/Celery with Raw Almond Butter
Avocado Toast
Popcorn (air popped)

Exercise/PT
I personally, do not recommend attempting to follow your usual exercise routine or to start a new one until you can do so without major repercussions. Any attempt to be overly physical may lead to a

flare up that would relegate you back to bed and ravage your hard-won mental stability.

I read on a blog from one of Dr. Feigenbaum's earlier patients that she was told to move as little as necessary for the first two years to ensure complete healing. I must admit that as soon as I was able, I moved quite a bit and would put myself into a flare up. Whether I took steps backwards by doing this is unclear to me. It was hard not to push myself too much, but I have learned that pushing is not the Tarlov/meningeal way. As your healing advances, you will need to try things and risk a flare up because you will not know what you can do until you try it. Something you could not do a month ago may be easy now. You cannot let the fear of a flare up prevent you from testing and reassessing your limits.

Dr. Feigenbaum recommends beginning physical therapy (although he did not use to) six months to one year following surgery. However, after meeting with a physical therapist and hearing the process, I opted out. I knew what I was capable of and if I went along with his suggested treatment, I would be in constant agonizing pain which I believed would set me back. During your recovery, it is so important you learn to listen to your own body and intuition. A doctor telling you to do something should not replace your own sense of what should be done. As your body recovers, you will know what you can handle and you will automatically move in the direction of what is physically possible for you.

Perhaps, you will face great judgement from your family and friends on this matter. I certainly did. I was told that I needed to learn to live with my pain and simply push through it. I was told that I needed to do physical therapy right away or I would never get better. I was told a great deal of things that made me feel isolated and confused. Your loved one's suggestions, no matter how misguided, are said from a place of love and helplessness.

The thing is, we are not recovering from a sport's injury, which does require physical therapy to rebuild muscle and tissue. Our nerves have been damaged and there is no amount of weightlifting or swimming that can speed the recovery of nerve function. Nerve damage does not allow for you to push through your pain and there is no real way to get on with your life until the pain has somewhat subsided. Imagine the pain of a severe toothache. Do you live with it? Do you grab a giant bag of beef jerky and go to town in hopes of strengthening the exposed nerve? Of course not, you call your dentist and beg for sweet relief or grab pliers and contemplate ripping the culprit out of your head yourself.

Nerve pain is not like other pain and neither is its healing protocol. Thank those that love you for wanting to help and let their suggestions roll off your back. You know what is best for you and you must honor your wisdom without feeling pressured by others. This is one of the great lessons from a Tarlov/meningeal cyst.

As you recover more and more, your body will naturally want to begin light stretches and you will walk as much as you can as soon as you can. Being bedridden for extended periods of time helps you to embrace your capabilities with vigor as they improve. Eventually, you can add in light hand weights and/or do wall pushups to help get your blood moving. Hot baths also speed up your heartrate and are considered an aerobic workout. This is important to utilize so that your pumping blood can circulate faster and help you to detox and recover. Some of you may be able to do much more than this. The point is to do what you can when you can and not a moment sooner.

A helpful habit to get into is to thank your body each time you can do something physical. Positive emotions are proven to speed recovery. When I do wall pushups, I say 'Thank You' with each one. This small habit can begin to create a new kind of relationship with your physical body that fosters love, gratitude and appreciation in a way that you may not have experienced prior to your diagnosis. Another gift.

Suggested Exercises
Isometrics
Wall Push-Ups
Static Positions
Stretching
Walking
Swimming

No bending, twisting, jumping, or running is suggested until you can do so without creating an intense flare-up. It is imperative you get in the habit of checking in with your body frequently. It has been suggested that if pain subsides after some rest following an activity, then it is a good amount of activity for the stage of healing you are at. If the pain persists, then you should reduce the activity until further healing has taken place. In this way, you can gauge what activity level is appropriate for you and what activities are still problematic. Once you recognize the offending motion/s, you can take steps to rectify it so that your life goes more smoothly. Perhaps, an additional EZ Reacher can solve your issues. Maybe you can buy a different piece of furniture or lay down while doing a task you normally do while sitting. Adjust your movements mindfully, so that you do not need to suffer more than is necessary in the healing process.

SURVIVING TARLOV

Chapter Eight
Emotional Support and Hope

In hindsight, I can see that my bigger battle was internal. I allowed myself to become entrenched in negativity, fear and darkness. I slipped into a void where no light could reach me for quite some time. Yet, there was light all around me. It took a lot of strength for me to reach out for it and it was imperative that I found a reason to push forward. For me, that reason was Damon and Lumen. I hope you have a reason just as strong to carry you through. This process is going to bring a lot of your shadows to the surface and you will be forced to face them or suffer the consequences. The beautiful part is, as soon as you do gather your courage, they will dissolve more quickly than you think.

Before this happened, I had terrible self-talk. I was constantly informing myself that I was not good enough, thin enough, or smart enough. I compared myself to other people that I thought had it figured out and felt jealousy and greed. I kept myself entrenched in shame for my past mistakes. I clung to areas where I believed I had gone wrong in life. Mostly, I wished myself to be completely and totally different than I was. Every time I had a mean thought about myself, my spirit would shrink back a bit more. Eventually, I lost all connection with my inner beauty and joy.

While going through this process, you will be faced with much fear and doubt. You might even terrify yourself by telling yourself that you will never recover, as I did. Eventually, this will become too much for you and you will learn that you may need to change how you talk to yourself. In my process, I noticed that I was slowly beginning to comfort myself. I would have a scary thought and I would catch myself counteracting the thought and telling myself that I was going to be okay. I started cheering myself on. I became my very best friend. This began a new and beautiful relationship with myself that continues to strengthen each day.

I realized that all the self-help books I had been reading had not worked because they were constantly sending the message that I needed help. They all laid out plans for how to better myself or change myself, which only sent the message that I was not good enough how I was. Then, when I could not adhere to the "improvement" plan, I turned on myself even further.

The truth is, once you love yourself, truly love yourself exactly as you are, you begin to improve any areas that actually need improvement effortlessly. You eat healthy because you love yourself. You treat yourself with kindness because you love yourself. You are patient with yourself because you love yourself. You do not rack up thousands in credit card debt because you love yourself. The list goes on and on, but you do not need to worry about any of it. Once you allow your innate self-love to take the forefront everything happens spontaneously and with joy.

Going through a traumatizing experience like a Tarlov/meningeal cyst opens a huge window of opportunity for you to release yourself from your old conditioned mindset and allows deep wounds to surface for healing. Being stripped down and vulnerable sets the groundwork for whole healing. There are resources that helped me with this process and they are:

Affirmation Wall
If you do not have any nice thoughts floating around in your head, borrow someone else's. Our minds are habitual, meaning they like to think the same things over and over. The good news is that you can exert your force and create new habits of thinking. It is vitally important that you find a way to be hopeful and kind to yourself.

One of the ways I achieved this was by gathering the most meaningful and inspirational quotes I could and taping them all over my bedroom wall. Every day, as I laid there, I stared at that wall and read all the affirmations and quotes repeatedly. I found it particularly helpful during a horrendous flare-up. Eventually, the positive thoughts on my wall moved into my mind and I was able to take them on as my own. The day I realized I no longer needed them, I got up and tore them all off with a smile.

Skype Therapy

At some point, it became clear to me that I needed mental and emotional help. I began having weekly Skype sessions with a therapist and it helped tremendously. She kept me focused on recovery and helped me to believe I would in fact recover. She encouraged me to get off Facebook, so that I would stop sinking into despair over my recovery not lining up with other's and stop taking on fears that did not belong to me. Our work together gave me something to focus on other than my physical limitations. I would spend a great deal of time journaling and working through issues. One of my biggest lessons was in managing my expectations of others.

During my initial recovery, I had expectations of how people would be there for me emotionally and physically. If they were not there for me in the ways I expected, then I allowed myself to feel betrayed and dismissed the ways they were showing up for me. My therapist helped me to understand that I needed to have clarity about what role each individual actually serves in my life. I was expecting comfort from people that were not good at comforting, but they were great at helping me forget my troubles for a while. Some people in your life will be good for entertainment, others will be good at motivation, some will be good at research, and some will be able to provide nurturing. Everyone serves an important function in your life and it is up to you to determine their actual role or else you will feel unnecessarily hurt by your own misplaced expectations.

Inspirational Reading

It is tempting to spend hours poring over horror stories of people's experiences with this disease, but it is certainly not helpful. Do yourself a favor and throw all that out the window. Read stories of triumph only. Find articles and books recounting stories of full recovery and overcoming all the odds.

You will be hard pressed to find too many stories in the area of TCD, but there are tons of other afflictions that are comparable. Any stories of individuals overcoming spinal injuries, amputations, shark attacks, etc. will remind you of how capable you and your body are. It will also demonstrate the ability to overcome nerve injuries in general. This task seems insurmountable from your viewpoint, but climb up my darling. A couple of my favorites are:

Miracle Man by **Morris Goodman**- This guy crashed his plane and ended up basically as a vegetable on a ventilator. No one believed he could ever recover, other than him, and that was enough. He set his mind to do it and eight months later he walked out of the hospital. This is a must read and truly highlights the importance of a perseverance mindset.

On My Own Two Feet by **Amy Purdy**- Amy somehow contracted meningitis and it quickly overtook her body, resulting in the loss of both of her legs, deformation to other areas of her body, and an eventual organ transplant. This is her story of how she overcame these limitations and went on to become a world-renowned snowboarder. It is incredibly inspirational and reminds us that there is the potential for a beautiful life after loss, if we can dare to reach for it.

Meditations
At times, you will find yourself in need of a mental break. Meditations abound on YouTube and cover a wide range of topics. Some ideas to get your search going are healing, recovery, pain management, positive thinking, and enlightenment. Whatever floats your boat is available for free.

Some of my favorite providers are Trigram Healing and Jason Stephenson. I like to listen to these when I am in the bath. I also have some purchased meditations that I rotate and highly recommend. Dr. Joe Dispenza and Kim Eng are a couple of my favorites and offer life changing potential.

Religion/Spirituality/Positive Psychology

No matter what your belief system is, now is the time to lean on and develop it further. You need all the help you can get and science has proven that those who have a strong belief system tend to recover more quickly. If you do not have spiritual or religious beliefs, then lean on science or positive psychology.

Chapter Nine
The Other Side

Here we are, at the end of this resource guide and probably the beginning of your journey. I sincerely hope that some of this information has and will help you through this. If there is one message I really hope to convey, it is this, you will recover. Your life will go on. You will find joy and happiness again. One day, your life will no longer be controlled by this diagnosis or your pain. I know how hard this is to believe and I know what you must go through to get there. I am deeply sorry that this has come to visit your doorstep. My heart does break for you and what you must endure, but it also shimmers with a silver lining. This is your hero's journey and you will come out on the other side a changed person. This too shall pass. This is but a long couple of chapters in your book of life. No one can tell you when things will get better, but they will.

One of the leaders of a Tarlov Facebook group was kind enough to call me one day and spent over an hour on the phone with me. She told me that she had been a part of the group for years and that in her experience, the majority would eventually recover with time. There are other things that factor into our recoveries, such as underlying conditions and overall physical, mental and emotional health. Which is another reason it is so important that we address all aspects of ourselves in the healing journey for the best possible outcome. We may not be alright in a month or year, but we will be alright.

It might surprise you in this moment to know that you have much to look forward to as a result of what you are currently enduring. In a haze of fear, anxiety, pain and confusion you may not be able to see how much growth and strength you are acquiring or the inner transformation that is taking place. You may not even be able to allow yourself to think into the future for fear of being disappointed. I was right there with you. In the beginning, every thought I could have about my future was tainted with a vison of myself on the sidelines forever. This will ease as your healing gets under way and you have verifiable proof that this will one day end. When you arrive at this point, you will certainly begin to look forward to being healed and returning to activity. However, there is much more waiting for you on the other side than simply being able to walk around a grocery store.

I believe there is a reason beyond our limited comprehension that this has happened to us. It changes us and infuses our lives with great love, gratitude and meaning. Before all this happened to me, I use to become so frustrated with my inner turmoil and lack of purpose that I would pray in tears for contentment. It was something I continually chased after through books and workshops, never quite hitting the mark. I can tell you that nothing brings more contentment than having everything you love stripped away from you and then being forced to slowly earn it back.

I wasted so much of my life trying to make it different then it was, erroneously believing that it was my environment that brought me such dis-ease. I continually tried to change myself and others around me to "fix" it. Once I lost everything that I had been attempting to run away from, I quickly realized that what I already had was all I ever needed. I did not miss the workshops and self-help books. I did not think a different career would somehow make me feel good enough. I did not think that if I changed my zip code everything would magically get better. I laid there in bed, day in and day out, in deep agonizing emotional and physical pain wanting nothing more than the life that was mine all along.

I discovered it was my thoughts making me discontent and I vowed to never let them trick me again into being ungrateful for the gift that is my existence. This is the greatest realization that comes from overcoming a Tarlov/meningeal cyst. Once you take your life back, you get to live it with love and appreciation. You no longer need outside validation or the materiality that permeates so much of our society. Some of the things you have to look forward to:

Self-Love

It is easy to focus on everyone else to the detriment of ourselves in everyday life. The problem arises when we become overly focused on the needs of others or begin to compare ourselves to them. Our minds are problem solvers and so if we have conditioned ourselves to live from the mind rather than the heart, we will always find some problem with ourselves that we feel compelled to dwell on or solve.

We tend to place parameters or conditions on whether we will love ourselves or not. We think we must first be a certain weight, have a certain job, a certain relationship, a certain house, a certain level of healing and so on before we can accept ourselves. When we are faced with something as traumatizing as a Tarlov/meningeal cyst, our minds go through many stages of grief that ultimately end with acceptance.

In our case, this is the acceptance of who we are, what matters to us in life and how we want to spend our precious time. As we heal and begin to make changes in our lives to match these revelations, it sends a signal to our hearts that we are now on our own side. From this, self-love begins to flourish.

Acceptance

Life is not always going to give you what you want or what you think you deserve. Life is just life. It plays itself out in a number of ways that are out of any of our individual control. There are too many moving parts in the scheme of things for you to protect yourself from things you would rather not experience. The good news is that we can learn not to see the natural unfolding of life as an enemy. This is again a trick of the mind that sees all things as a problem to be solved.

Life is happening as it is happening. What may be considered good to one person is detrimental to another. Losing any sense of control of our lives while going through this, is at first a source of great suffering. However, with prolonged suffering, a new quality begins to emerge. That quality is acceptance. It is the precursor to surrender.

You are not surrendering your hopes and dreams. You learn to surrender all of the thoughts in your mind that keep you in a state of suffering. The thoughts that create doubt and fear must go if you are to find peace. Your analytical mind cannot save you from your pain. To the contrary, it may only add to it as it creates the illusion of control. With this disease, we are along for the ride and all we can do is help ourselves and love ourselves through it with complete acceptance.

Gratitude

It is hard to have gratitude when your mind keeps you focused on the future. It is tempting to reach out ahead of ourselves and grab onto a goal that we think might bring us closer to feeling okay on the inside. However, the reason we do not feel okay on the inside to start with is because we are rejecting what we have and reaching for something we do not.

This creates a deep experience of lack in ourselves and our lives. If we believe we are lacking in what we need or want, then it becomes difficult to see what is right in front of us. This Tarlov/meningeal cyst experience takes away our ability to work towards any thing other then getting out of pain and recovering our mobility. We begin to see all the wanting and reaching as futile and painful. This helps us to begin to look around and appreciate what is here now. We can begin to clearly see all that we have to be grateful for and our love intensifies. When we begin to count our blessings, gratitude and contentment grows.

Presence

When you are experiencing pain and suffering, the mind can be a dangerous place to be. It might even add to your pain by dwelling on it. It could tell you that you will never be better. Perhaps, it shows you images of missing out on your whole life over and over. Being locked into that dark energy will undoubtedly force you to seek refuge elsewhere.

Where is elsewhere? Elsewhere is now. The present moment. The reality that is occurring, outside of your thoughts about it. Spiritual teacher Eckhart Tolle often asks individuals who are trapped in fear to evaluate what is wrong right now, in this moment. Often, the thing we are fearful of is not actually happening aside from a mental movie playing out in our heads. This helps you to focus on the truth.

Yes, you are in a great deal of pain. That is true. You should take steps to help alleviate some of your pain. That is your reality. To get lost in fears over surgery or whether you will ever heal are thoughts that are not based in your current reality of what is happening. When surgery is imminent, then you can deal with those emotions in that moment. You do not need to live through that fear repeatedly when it is only happening once.

The truth is that you cannot see into the future and so you do not know what your healing process is going to look like and neither does anyone else who you might seek validation from about the recovery process. If you are going to use your imagination at all to visualize a future you cannot know, then I would recommend imagining a positive outcome.

Faith

This whole situation is a roller coaster in faith. At first, you may become angry with God, the universe, or life itself. Any faith you may have had, may begin to waiver or be suppressed as the feelings of self-pity build up. This will pass and your faith will return with a reverence you have never known before.

You will no longer be living based on dogma provided from other's interpretations. You will have gone through a process that has given you direct inner wisdom and a strength that comes from the experience of being cared for by something bigger than yourself. You will be forced, in a sense, to develop a greater faith in God, the Universe, the Light or whatever you wish to call it.

In the end, once your pain begins to subside, you will slowly begin to see the lessons you have learned in action. You will have been transformed by this and the silver lining and purpose of it all will reveal itself through you. You were meant for something great and this is going to push you towards that path. In my opinion, that is the whole reason this has happened to us.

In Conclusion

I could not have known 11 years ago what all would transpire. For many years, I wished to go back to that fateful day when I tripped over the bloodhound and just step on her instead. For a long time, I erroneously believed if that fall had been avoided, then I could have avoided all the pain and immense suffering. The truth is, I cannot know what would have happened and if it had not been the fall, it would likely have been something else. It was simply part of my path in life to go through this. Just as it is yours. Regrets, blame, resentment and anger will eventually fall away and the true beauty of who you are and what you are meant to do in this life will replace it. I wish I could come to you and hold your hand and whisper all the secrets I now know will be revealed to you in time. I wish I could show you the person you will be once you have won the war. In the end, you will be totally and completely free. I want you to know that I love you with all my heart and I will be waiting here for you on the other side.

It Couldn't Be Done
By Edgar Albert Guest

Somebody said that it couldn't be done
But he with a chuckle replied
That "maybe it couldn't," but he would be one
Who wouldn't say so till he'd tried.
So he buckled right in with the trace of a grin
On his face. If he worried he hid it.
He started to sing as he tackled the thing
That couldn't be done, and he did it!

Somebody scoffed: "Oh, you'll never do that;
At least no one ever has done it;"
But he took off his coat and he took off his hat
And the first thing we knew he'd begun it.
With a lift of his chin and a bit of a grin,
Without any doubting or quiddit,
He started to sing as he tackled the thing
That couldn't be done, and he did it.

There are thousands to tell you it cannot be done,
There are thousands to prophesy failure,
There are thousands to point out to you one by one,
The dangers that wait to assail you.
But just buckle in with a bit of a grin,
Just take off your coat and go to it;
Just start in to sing as you tackle the thing
That "cannot be done," and you'll do it.

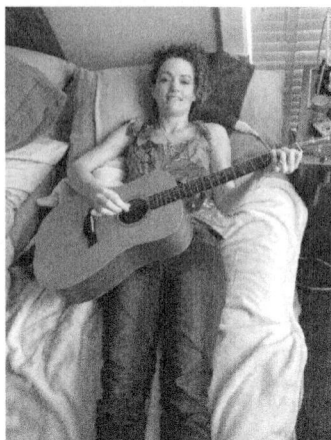

Practicing Guitar

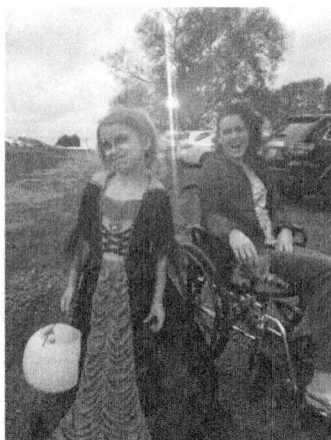

Halloween - 14 Months Post-Op

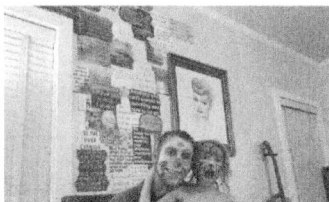

My Affirmation Wall

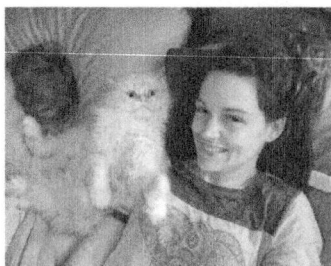

Bed Buddies - Zeus and Lumen

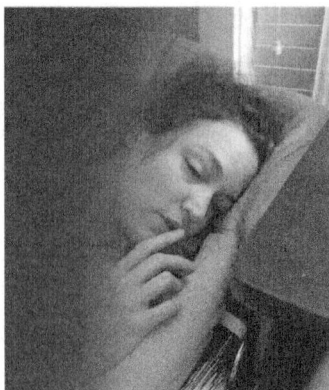

The Reality of a Flare

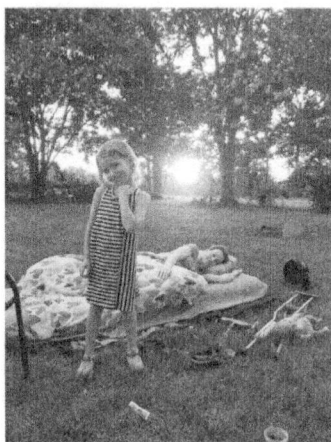

Life from the Ground

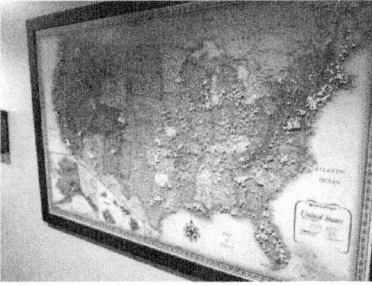

USA Map of Feigenbaum Patients

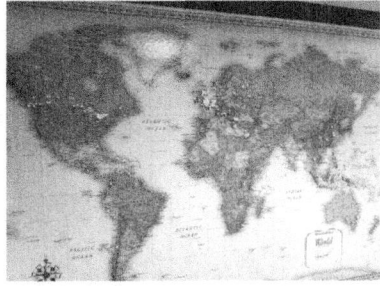

World Map of Feigenbaum Patients

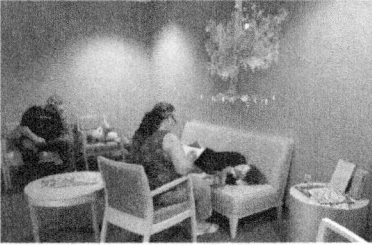

Consultation with Dr. Feigenbaum

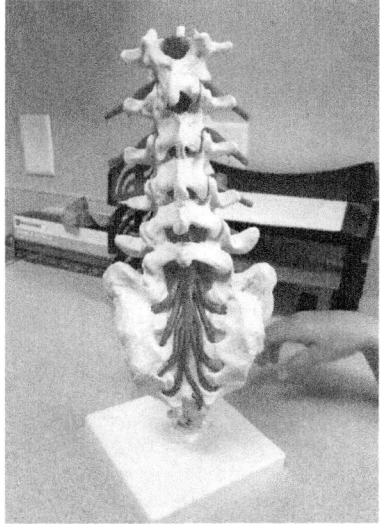

Model of Sacral Nerves

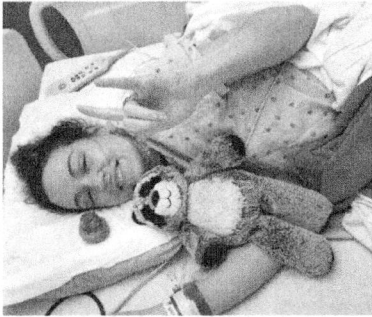

Letting Lumen know I was OK

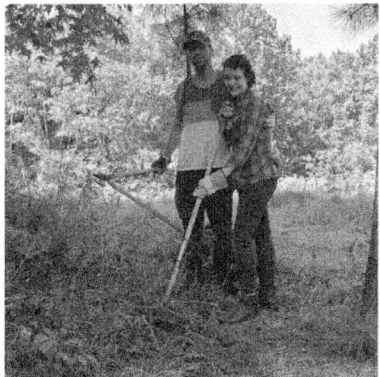

Placing Pin at Follow-Up

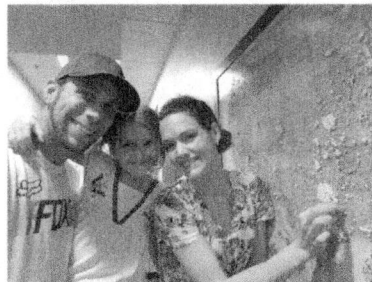

Clearing Land - 26 Months Post-Op

My nervous system vibrates with healing energy from head to toe.

ABOUT THE AUTHOR

Sheryl Bacon Jones is a published children's book author and her work has appeared in Conscious Zine and Mary Jane's Farm Magazine. She is also the Creative Director for the world's largest online school for activity professionals. She has authored and taught numerous bestselling continuing education courses for improving the lives of residents and the betterment of living conditions within the long-term care industry. She has a Bachelor's in Human Sciences and is working towards her PhD in Conscious Centered Living. In the summer of 2009, she began the long journey of discovery and recovery from a meningeal cyst. This entire process transformed her life in ways that she is still evolving from. Her areas of interests include health, nutrition, spirituality, love and empathy. She can be found with her husband, daughter and ragdoll, Puddles, somewhere in the woods of Texas.

You can find her at www.sharingsheryl.com

Have a success story you want to share? Let's help others heal through hope together. Big or small, send them all to sheryl@sharingsheryl. Thank you.

Printed in Great Britain
by Amazon

47355232R00040